Table of Contents

Introduction:

The art of presenting one's own argument can often take time to develop, and even longer to master. Many dread the thought of public speaking as developing original arguments and counter arguments can be daunting. Thinking of discussion topics spontaneously in front of an audience is intimidating for most individuals. However, what if one was to take away the audience and replace speech with writing, would that be slightly less confronting? Perhaps for some, but written forms of speeches and argumentative pieces in the form of essays can be equally daunting for others. Either way, in order to pass the GAMSAT the great obstacle to your medical career, one is bound to prepare for the daunting task of perfecting essays unless one wishes to approach it unprepared.

An essay is often compared to a debate or a public speech for an audience, although unlike debates, an essay prefers the written word. This could potentially be a much less frightening exercise as it allows an individual to re-organise thoughts and erase paragraphs that don't sound convincing. With a strictly regulated time limit however, covering mistakes or erasing discussion points can become difficult, and some would argue that writing an essay is no less difficult.

The word essay is known to invoke a certain apprehension among students not unlike the GAMSAT. To prevent such daunting experience from overwhelming a candidate, it is important to understand why individuals become uneasy when asked to write an essay.

The main three reasons include:

1. Not understanding what an essay is or how to structure it
2. Inability to develop convincing arguments
3. Lack of preparation and research

The second and third reasons are well addressed in this book and should be part of your preparation/research in your journey of GAMSAT essay preparation. This essay collection will also provide an insight into the preparation of my own GAMSAT journey as an undergraduate.

The first reason however is often the greatest obstacle. Essay writers are often not familiar with the structure of an essay. A 19th century sailor would not dare to sail too far away from the harbour without being able to navigate the stars. Therefore, prior to all preparation, the most important step is to understand how to navigate the essay structure as proficiently as a 19th century sailor could navigate the stars. Only then can an individual truly tailor an essay to address the essay question. The greatest reassurance is that it is not particular difficult to navigate the essay structure, and once an individual comprehends its structure; writing great essays will become effortless. However, prior to writing great essay, it is important to understand what the GAMSAT is and why it requires individuals to write two essays.

What is the GAMSAT:

Graduate Australian Medical School Admission Test, otherwise known as the GAMSAT is an exam developed and co-ordinated by the Australian Council for Education Research (ACER) developed to rank participants based on their performance. The GAMSAT is a standardised exam intended to evaluate an individual's capacity for tertiary graduate education in the medical and healthcare university courses. It is an exam required for the entry to all post-graduate medical school in Australia except for one (Sydney University), along with other universities in Ireland and United Kingdom. The GAMSAT is also required for some post-graduate courses in the field of dentistry and optometry courses. The exam has three sections, each focused on separate skills and is designed to appraise the participants critical thinking and communication skills.

The first section of the GAMSAT includes 75 questions in a multiple-choice form based mainly the field of humanities and social sciences. The questions in this section are based on various stimulus provided in the form of news-articles, paragraphs from a novel, images as well as other historical and ahistorical excerpts. A total of 100 minutes is permitted to answer the questions in section 1 in order to evaluate how well participants perform in critical thinking and reasoning based on the stimulus.

Section 2 employs a very different format and it is what this collection is focused on. The exam dedicates 60 minutes to evaluate how well participants master their written communication in the form of essays or creative writings. Two essays/writings are required to respond to quotes provided in the exam, and participants language, grammar, content and organisation are all assessed by examiners. More information about GAMSAT section 2 is included in later chapters.

A further 110 multiple choice questions are found in the third section. These questions need to be completed in less than 3 hours (170 minutes); the equivalent of 90 seconds per question. The short duration provided for each question is one of the main reasons the 3rd section of the GAMSAT is dreaded by many participants. A further reason is due to the heavy emphasis on biological and physical sciences, and this section is intended to assess reasoning, interpretation, critical thinking and problem-solving abilities of participants. It is often an advantage to have a science background for section 3, however, many of the questions are based on interpretation of scientific passages and diagrams, and skills in critical thinking will prove to be valuable in such settings.

Medicine:

If GAMSAT is such a dreadful experience, why do people sit the exam? The simple answer is Medicine. Although the GAMSAT is utilised as an entry exam for several disciplines including dentistry and other health degrees, the majority who attempt the GAMSAT, opt to apply for medicine. There are plenty criticisms of the nature of the GAMSAT, including that it is unnecessary difficult and lengthy. Many individuals also claim the exam does not reflect candidate's true abilities. Some arguments are valid in that some candidates simply don't perform as well under exam conditions relative to real life practical problem solving. However, despite the difficulty and length of the GAMSAT, it currently entails an integral part of selecting for future doctors and dentists. Even if the material in GAMSAT does not reflect real life medical situation, it certainly assesses an individual's ability to think critically in stressful situations. The essay section also evaluates an individual's ability to express their ideas in a simple, but also free flowing direction that make it easy for readers to comprehend.

Despite the challenge GAMSAT place on candidates, if medicine is their passion, it certainly is worth dedicating great amount of time to achieve a competitive percentile. A career in medicine will take individuals inside the human body on the operating table, in the mind of individuals in a psychiatric hospital and make future doctors a witness to the most joyful, as well as the most painful events of patient's lives. It is difficult to imagine another career that offers such great privilege to be trusted with their clients/patient's life. No matter how difficult one may think entering medical school is, it certainly offers a lot of reward in return if medicine is the goal of the applicant. This essay collection is designed to assist applicants into entering medical school

The Essay collection:

This essay collection does not consist of perfect essays, but rather examples of essays that were written by myself in preparation of my own GAMSAT. Having successfully passed the GAMSAT and entered medical school, a collection of non-polished essays completed under time restrictions are published in this book designed. This approach has been purposely chosen to assist future applicants with an insight into the preparation of a previous applicant and to learn from common errors. Errors that have been repeated several times previously and which have had a negative impact on the overall score of essays. If an individual is confident in writing essays and simply want to read through the examples, please skip to the 'Essay Collection' section.

Many writers find essay writing complex at first, and this is partly because there are many overlapping definitions of what an essay truly is. The varying definitions become rather complicated as essays do not share a particular format such as letters. The lack of a universal accepted definition of an essay is often responsible for the difficulty in mastering essays. However, the lack of definition can also be its strength, as in the hand of an experienced author, the format can be adjusted depending on its audience.

A simple definition proposes that an essay is a document which includes argumentative writing with the aim of convincing the reader of a certain viewpoint. However, an essay can take many shapes and can be tailored to its audience. A well-rehearsed essay writer understands this and can take full advantage of it. For less experienced writers, the basic format remains a powerful tool, the question remains, what is a basic essay?

A basic essay is an argument either in the affirmative or negative relative to the essay question consisting of an introduction, paragraph and conclusion. Even though one can entertain both sides on the argument without choosing a firm position; this can often seem indecisive or non-committal. Such a stance can be well suited for an advanced writer, however, for less experienced writers, such a position can be difficult to discuss adequately.

Once a viewpoint is established, the essay structure consists of an introduction, paragraphs and a conclusion. The introduction is designed to offer the audience an understanding of the position of the writer and an outline into the arguments that will be established without listing the arguments. The introduction is then followed by paragraphs with and most GAMSAT essays written with 3-5 paragraphs.

A paragraph can be thought of a mini essay in that it has an introduction, body and conclusion, however, essential differences remain. It is essential that each paragraph has only one argument/point to prove. In other words, each paragraph should only contain a single statement/point in support of the wider position the author establishes with the remaining of the paragraph aimed at supporting the paragraph's point. Therefore, an essay that is in support of making it compulsory for all primary school children to have a laptop could have a paragraph with a strong statement. An example of could state the following; "In a future with advancing technology, a young adult who is not well versed with using a laptop will struggle to find employment". This statement will need to be supported by evidence in the form of an example, quote or statistic. An explanation will follow the statement and the evidence to further clarify the authors position. This will then lead to the conclusion of the paragraph by linking the explanation back to the original essay question to highlight why the author holds a specific view relative to the essay question. This basic structure is also known as the PEEL paragraph, PEEL standing for point, example, explanation and link. Following such structure can be considered safe, however, with more experience one can also customize it depending on the type of structure they write.

Finally, after all the paragraphs are written, it is important to conclude the essay. The final conclusion is not all that different from the introduction as it also outlines the essay's key points and reaffirms the position that was established in the introduction. Unlike the introduction however, the conclusion must not only outline the main points of the essays, but also summarise them. It can further afford an explanation into why some people may argue in opposition and the reasoning why the opposing view is flawed or a less credible position to hold.

The introduction, paragraphs and essay are the main composition of the basic essay structure. However, more is required than what is written on the paper. The few minutes prior and post writing an essay is of crucial importance, and knowledgeable essay writers will utilise every second they have. Most essay writers do not utilise the few minutes prior or post essay writing effectively. This mistake is often labelled as the beginner's error. However, many experienced writers also make the same mistake. A few minutes set aside prior to the essay writing can give the author just enough time to establish the position he/she will hold and their main points. If an individual is planning to have three paragraphs, it is essential to have three strong and unique points to argue. Jumping into an essay without those key arguments can make even the introduction a difficult part to write, after all, how can the audience understand the position of the author, when the author has not spent more than a few seconds to establish their own position on the essay question. It is also equally important to leave a few minutes after writing the essay to have a brief overlook at the essay, ensuring that what is written portray the same message the author had meant for it to depict.

GAMSAT Section 2:

The essay collection in this book focuses on section 2 of the GAMSAT which involves two written components. An hour is provided for the two components with an additional 5 minutes reading time. Section 2 is the only written part of the exam and it is the section where participants can truly demonstrate their true understanding of the human sentiment. It requires participants to formulate a persuasive essay/written component twice, with only 30minute allocation for each writing. In such short period of time, it is essential to use the 5 minutes reading time to good effect for both reading and planning purposes. Due to the time restrictions, it is also essential that part of the planning purpose is conducted prior to the exam. In the following pages, section two will be further broken down into several parts in order to better understand better what is required by applicants.

Section 2: part A:

- Surrounds socio-cultural issues and themes
- Essays with strong arguments are essential
- No reflection is required

Section 2, part A requires participants to write an essay similar in structure to those taught in school. These are essays with basic structures comprising of an introduction, several paragraphs and a conclusion. Five quotes are given in part A, and the applicant's task is to choose one or more quotes to base their essay on. If a candidate finds essay writing complicated, then it's often easier to stay with a single quote and to either firmly agree or firmly disagree with the quote/statement chosen. This part requires an individual to put forward their strongest arguments for a point and convince the examiner of their viewpoint. The stronger and more organised the better the essay, particularly when combined with a logical flow of ideas. The writing component of Part A basically require a strong and convincing style of writing for the audience to be convinced of the author's views in an essay format.

Section 2: part B:

- Involves personal/social issues and themes
- Arguments are less important
- Reflection and creativeness are imperative

Section 2, part B differ greatly from part A in the type of quotes candidates can choose from and the style of writing it demands. The quotes in part B are often not argumentative in nature and involve personal issues such as love and family. It requires an individual to bring out the artistic side and place a touch of creativeness in their writing. No debating is required in part B, but rather reflection and imagination is what is most sought after. The type of writing required in part B enables individuals to show their flair and place personal touches in their writings. This creativeness often requires individuals to find their own unique writing style and most would agree that this section requires more practice than part A.

Essays Collection:

In both parts of section 2, candidates are given 5 quotes to choose one or multiple quotes for their written piece. Candidates are given 5 minutes reading time to read, choose which quotes to include and if time permits also plan the essay. For Part A Essays, it is essential that individuals begin their essays by defining the keywords in the quotes and including those keywords in the essay. Practicing this method enables the examiner to better understand the author's interpretation of the quote/topic and even more importantly, safeguards candidates from wavering on their prospective arguments. It is critical to establish definitions prior to starting any essay, and although it is not required, it is considered excellent preparation to include definitions in practice essays. Including definitions is an important training exercise to establish an individual's understanding of the main words in the quotes provided. Often the importance of establishing definitions is ignored by many, resulting in less consistent arguments with no understanding of the quotes/topic established. It is important to note that definitions do not require to be consistent with mainstream or dictionary definition, but rather one that is relative to the stimulus provided and what the author interprets them to mean.

Once the definitions are established, it is important to establish the points the candidate wishes to make in their paragraphs. It is essential to remember that each paragraph will require a distinct point. Developing points after establishing a definition is essential as each point will need to be consistent with the author's understanding of the quote and topic. It is also important to establish points prior to writing the essay, as it is difficult to write an introduction to an argumentative essay if a candidate is uncertain of his/her main points of the argument. It may seem like a time-consuming method, but it is critical to follow this method to write a strong, convincing and logical essay from beginning to end. Candidates will find it much more time consuming if any corrections in the essay is required or if they believe that one of their stronger points were not included. Practicing this method of establishing definitions and arguments prior to writing an essay may be very time consuming initially, but this is an art that could be reduced to less than a minute with sufficient practice. Any more than five minutes will place writers in severe disadvantage as it will take up a significant portion of the total time allocated for writing the essay. With sufficient practice, experienced essay writers may even be able to follow the proposed method and be ready to write their essay plan within the five-minute reading time.

Another mental exercise for type A essays is the ability to entertain, even if only for a brief moment, both sides of the argument. As part of essay practice, candidates should practice writing both a short thesis and an anti-thesis consisting of opposing viewpoints and arguments. Although the counterarguments to the chosen viewpoint would rarely change the mind of the author, it certainly allows for both sides to be entertained and enables enhanced arguments. This approach may not be possible during the GAMSAT as it would take away valuable exam time, however, the exercise of developing counterarguments to the established viewpoint is intended to train the mind to entertain both sides of the argument. This method would make the audience appreciate that the individual has accounted for the opposing view, making the established arguments even more comprehensive and convincing.

Type B essay/writing task is different from that of task A. Task B does not require a writer to adopt a strict structure and permits for creativeness and personal touch in the writing piece. The quotes or statements provided for applicants are different from that of task A in that they invoke emotions. Most quotes or statement involve a personal/social issue which demands reflection and an emotional insight. The example essays provided do not follow a specific structure, but rather focuses on the themes and aim to invite the readers to reflect and question a certain theme. There is no right or wrong in task B essay as long as reflection and creativeness are involved. Some of the example essays are written as ordinary essays which is acceptable but will not warrant an excellent grade. However, despite the lack of structure, these writings can also be planned prior to being written with established definitions, thesis and anti-theses along with ideas for each paragraph.

The following essays are written as examples of what to expect in the GAMSAT exam.

Type A Essays:

The science of today is the technology of tomorrow

Keywords: Science, today, technology, tomorrow

Definitions:

Science: The study of nature which is limited by time and space

Today: The present time.

Technology: equipment and software produced and developed based on engineering and applied sciences.

Tomorrow: Anytime in the future.

Affirmative/Thesis: Current technology is based on scientific discoveries of the past, which is a great prediction that future technology will be based on current scientific discoveries.

Negative/Anti-thesis: Although some of the technology we have today is based on previous scientific discoveries, however patterns of the past not a certain predictor of future technological discoveries.

Author's perspective: Affirmative

Title: Science of today; the technology of tomorrow.

Since the very first step taken by humankind, discoveries of the natural world have been made and technology have soon imitated these findings. Although the modern scientific method may only be a few centuries old, the observation of nature has been responsible for great advances in technology since time immemorial. The fields of physics, chemistry and biology have been particularly important in the development of technology which we rely on a daily basis. Without these fields of sciences, we would likely still be travelling with horse carriages and sending handwritten letters by ships across the world. There is little doubt when exploring examples of today's technology that many have derived from previous scientific advances, a reflection that that the science of today will certainly be the technology of tomorrow.

Perhaps the first scientific enquiry of humankind was the observation of both flora and fauna. The study of zoology was certainly important for the first humans to develop strategies to safely co-exist with surrounding animals. For millennia, the feat of flying which birds possessed was an impossibility for humankind. The science of zoology spent great efforts at marvelling and studying the amazing exploit of flying even before Da Vinci's blueprint for the first helicopter. His desire to fly was shared by many throughout history, and this desire was well expressed in many scientific studies and drawings. However, much later the wright brothers conquered the ability to fly, with an aircraft based on their intricate study of birds flying. The wright brothers may only have designed a wooden plane at the time, but it possessed the tree axis system which enabled aircraft to remain airborne, technology which is still found in modern aircrafts. Despite flying only for 12 seconds over a distance of 36 metres, it was the beginning of humankind challenging nature on the design of who could manufacture the most efficient flying machine. Although the first aircraft was based on centuries of scientific enquiry and did not resemble modern aircraft, the developers were certain further science would produce more efficient aircrafts. This proved to be true, and more advanced aircrafts were produced. Aircrafts developed in accordance with latest discoveries in the field of physics and based on the science of zoology continued to offer us the technology we have today and will continue to offer us more advanced aircrafts in the future.

The camera was based on the scientific study of the eye. Since the beginning of history, the only way to record visual surroundings was through art and storytelling. However, through the extensive study of human and animal eyes, science have been finally found the answers to replicate such amazing machinery. Today's digital camera can be found everywhere, including our phones, computes, CCTV, our pocket cameras and professional DSLR cameras. These devices store our most precious memories, and their clarity continues to improve constantly. They are amazing at replicating what the human eye has been doing since the beginning of time. However, there has been great criticism regarding the design flaws of the human eye, one most notable critic is Richard Dawkins who claims that many other animals such as the eagle has much better sight than humans. However, the human eye has some great supporters in the scientific world which will remind that healthy human eyes have 500 megapixels in clarity and has their own automatic zoom, focus and shutter functions. No camera has clarity anywhere close to 500 megapixels, and there does not appear to be any sign of any camera with even 100 megapixels being developed anytime soon. What critics like Dawkins fail to mention is that both the analogue and the digital cameras were designed by imitating many of the features of the human eye. The biological field of ophthalmology have led to great understanding of how the human vision works, and great emphasis is placed in scientific circles to better understand how the eye effortlessly make all these features work. The science or more specifically the biology of the human eye have provided us with the technology we have today which continues to advance tomorrow's world.

The scientific study to understand projectile motion have led to some awe-inspiring technology such as space shuttles and satellites. Other technologies such as missiles and nuclear bombs are also impressive, although less beneficial to humankind. The scientific field of projectile motion have enabled us to better understand gravity and also advanced our technology in establishing satellites which make GPS devices possible. It would be difficult to imagine a world without GPS technology today, nor a world where we were yet to send out space shuttles to the moon or discover the boundaries of our solar system. Technology which have made a greater impact than GPS is hard to identify, but the technology of flying has also been extensively advanced through the study of projectile motion. Therefore, it can be easily observed that what was once simply the study of physics and projectile motion have become the technology of tomorrow. Extensive research is currently being advanced in the physical studies of projectile motion and its associated disciplines such as aerodynamics and jet engines that one could only predict what today's physics will bring forward in tomorrow's technology. One thing is certain, today's physics will be a more imposing version of tomorrow's technology

Fleming, the famous Belgian microbiologist discovered penicillin in the petri-dish, however the ability to utilise the discovery evaded him. Further advances in pharmacology resulted in Australian pharmacologist Howard Florey to extract penicillin which have saved hundreds of thousands of lives. The simple petri dish which was designed to make a haven for bacteria to grow would prove to be the salvation of millions, if not billions in the future. In the early 20th century, a simple infection such as mild pneumonia could claim the life of many individuals. A simple cut or a drink from contaminated water could be a life sentence for many. However, Fleming would soon make such life sentences a thing of the past with the advent of antibiotics. Although borne out of an accident, the inability for bacteria to grown in the vicinity of the substance called penicillin would lead to extensive advanced technology of anti-infective medications including oral and intravenous antibiotics. Although penicillin came as a result of an accident, modern antibiotics have derived from the use of technology which analyse the receptors of bacteria and formulate antibiotics to target specific receptors. The technology involved in the formulation and delivery of modern antibiotics are a result of the science of yesterday. The science of yesterday has given rise to the technology of producing antibiotics. Further advances in the field of microbiology and pharmacology will better prepare us for the pandemics of the future.

Although it is difficult to predict what technology will derive from today's science, past scientific advances have certainly led to technology which we have benefited greatly from. Past scientific advances in all scientific fields have contributed to technology we could not live without. The technology of flying, the camera, space technology and other medical advances are all notable technologies based on previous scientific discoveries. Based on these great technological achievements from previous scientific advances, it is reasonable to conclude that today's science will lead to greater technology tomorrow.

"The mother of Revolution is Crime and Poverty" Aristotle

Definitions:

Revolution: the forcible overthrow government or social order in favour of a new system.

Crime: an act which is considered illegal by the constitute a person is located in, and is punishable by law

Poverty: is a state having minimal or no wealth or being in a state of inferior quality

Mother: the entity or source that gives rise to a new creation/society/individual

Affirmative/Thesis: Social failures found in revolutions often stem from an incompetent governing body. A governing body which fails to provide for its citizens adequately provides the basis for a revolution. The inadequacies from poverty and crime against humanity have often been the main reasons for uprisings and revolutions of the past. Thus, it would be safe to say the state of poverty and acts of crimes could and should be labelled as the mothers of revolution.

Negative/Anti-thesis: Revolutions are often thought of as political acts and are not necessarily related to corruption. A large number of revolutions resulted in greater crime, corruption and often living standard became worse as a result. Famous examples include the communist revolution of Russia in 1917 and the Nazi revolution in Germany in 1933. These examples both highlight two systems where both crime and poverty increased in both frequency and intensity.

Position of author: Affirmative

Title: "The mother of revolution is crime and poverty"

Since the dawn of human civilisation, revolutions have been utilised to replace governments to bring in a new social order. The beginnings of such revolutions have often been sparked by government failures and their inability to provide for the general public. Not being provided with wealth or safety, many citizens have reason to ask for or perhaps even actively pursue a change in their governing bodies. Although it is true that many factors can and have contributed to revolutions of the past, no factors have been as potent as crime and poverty. So potent are crime and poverty to bring about a revolution that even ancient historians like Aristotle recognised their influence and labelled them the "mother of revolution".

In every society, there are issues which make citizens frustrated, however, two particular issues that have people up in arms are crime and poverty. These two issues appear to be unforgivable in that they rob the nation of wealth and safety, providing citizens with little reason not wish for change. Most notable contemporary examples where crime and poverty brought about a revolution is the African nation of Libya under Gaddafi. Libya was known to have vast natural resources, and yet the nation was plagued with poverty and rampant crime. Corruption and lack of planning by people in positions of power led to high levels of crime, poverty and in the aforementioned examples even civil war. Countries like Libya among others provide a good example on how a corrupt government limit the safety and wealth of its citizens and lead to a society full of crime and poverty. The Libyan revolution was justified for a large number of reasons, but it was evident that the mother of these reasons were high levels of crime and poverty.

Certain revolutions are believed to be caused by nationalism and desire of self-governance with crime and poverty only as a second though. However, it can be appreciated that although a nation may be relatively free from crime and poverty, certain groups within a nation may not enjoy the same privileges relative to the rest of the population. A notable example from history is that of the former republic of Yugoslavia in 1991. Yugoslavia was often thought of as a relatively peaceful and stable nation where levels of crimes and poverty were relatively low in comparison to most other nations. However, the majority of wealth remained firmly in the hand of the Serbian part of the population, and much less were granted for the people of Croatia, Slovenia and Macedonia. The non-Serbian population of Yugoslavia were experiencing much greater levels of crime and poverty, and it was not long until a revolution was in full motion and Yugoslavia would disintegrate into many different nations. Although this particular revolution did have a component of nationalism, and other political motives, the issues of crime and poverty were certainly strong underlying factors.

Several revolutions have also been waged against the ruling class by its citizens for the vast difference in wealth between the ruling class and ordinary citizens. The poverty faced by ordinary citizens in middle eastern nation when the upper and ruling class have some of the world's wealthiest individuals in the world is nothing short of a crime against humanity. Several middle eastern nations had a change of rulers throughout the middle east in the previous years, and several more privileges have been offered to the working class. The governments of Yemen and Syria have been put to the test as their citizens no longer want to see their children die of starvation while watching their rulers enjoy all the luxuries in life. It appears that crime and poverty is not accepted by society and if it persists, will naturally lead to further revolutions.

Revolutions, or the forcible overthrow of status quo is result of several reasons, however, crime and poverty are often the greatest drivers of revolution. Many motives can be attributed to revolutions, however, as in all the previous examples it is notable that the common denominator remains crime and poverty. It appears that although other reasons can act as powerful motivators, however, in isolation these reasons remain only motivators and are unable to sustain a revolution. Therefore, it can be appreciated that as Aristotle suggested, crime and poverty are often the source, or in other words the mother of revolutions.

Technology may be beneficial, but at the expense of social capital

Definitions:

Technology: equipment and software produced and developed based on engineering and applied sciences.

Beneficial: resulting in good or beneficial circumstances.

Expense: the fee incurred when acquiring goods and/or services.

Social Capital: the effective functioning of individuals in a community or groups through relationships, shared identity, tradition, level of trust and co-operation among such individuals.

Affirmative/Thesis: Technology have proven to be beneficial, and the industrial revolution have been a great example to economic growth. However, with technology, many communities have noticed a loss in social connection and sense of community.

Negative/Anti-theses: Technology has been both beneficial and has brought people together. Prior to the telegram, the telephone and the internet, it would have taken greater than a month for relatives to hear from one another across the Atlantic Ocean.

Author's perspective: Affirmative

Title: The cost of technology

It is not possible to deny the positive outcome of technology throughout history as its benefits are obvious. Ranging from the time of Sumerians who invented the wheel to they modern day civilisation who invented the internet, technology seems to gradually become a more permanent part of our lives.

Changes forced upon us by technology will most certainly influence the lives of individuals in numerous aspects and is often found consuming valuable time which in the past was spent with family, friends and the community. Technology may even have a greater social cost than one might have anticipated if left unchecked. Michael Harrington stated that "if there is technological advance without social advance, there is, almost automatically an increase in human misery". Keeping in mind how accessible technology is to people of all ages in the western world, social advance is not, and may never be able to keep up with the rate of new technology.

Considering the large numbers of people on social websites such as Facebook and Google +, it is becoming increasingly difficult finding time for physical interactions. People of all ages are spending an increasing number of hours on their electronic gadgets and internet throughout the day. Everyday activities such as shopping, and banking are gradually being replaced by a few clicks on the computer. Technology has become "the science of arranging life so one does not need to experience it". This quote highlights the problem of technology as it replaces the social aspects of life. A growing number of questions have been raised about the youth's ability to socialise and their ability to communicate amidst the overwhelming ability of technology to replace the experience of face to face communication. The further our lives are entwined with technology; the less time and effort individuals will place of physical interaction and the building of social capital.

The internet is nothing but a vast ocean full of information which has proven to be difficult to regulate. Such information has served the current generation in more ways than what could possibly have been imagined a century ago. The possibility of communication with anyone in the world within a couple seconds have made this world highly efficient and contributed greatly to the high living standard that citizens of the world are enjoying today. In a large number of circumstances, it is the technological advances in laboratories, hospitals, and in our homes that have reduced human misery, and increased our ability to truly experience life like never before. Never has it been possible to travel around the world within days, shop from the comfort of your living room or to communicate with friends and family in different countries. The great benefits the human race has gained from what technology has provided is substantial however, it still remains to be seen if technology can replace the simpler things in life. Simple things such as the human touch, the helping hand or even a simple smile, acts which social capital depends on.

Although it might seem that technology has taken a great toll on social life, the true benefit and advantages of technology must be considered. There have been examples of advances in social capital in communication, however, it has proven to take a personal toll in face to face experiences. Technology have made great stride in increasing the wealth and productiveness of the world; however, it has also pushed families and friends further apart. Being driven further apart, there has been noticed a loss of social capital resulting in less traditions, social congregations and community gatherings.

"It is better that ten guilty persons escape, than one innocent suffers" William Blackstone

Definitions:

Guilty persons: an individual who is responsible for a specified wrongdoing.

Escape: the action of breaking free from imprisonment.

Innocent: an individual who has been incorrectly accused or charged with a wrongdoing.

Suffers: being subjected to an unpleasant experience.

Thesis: A community is built upon men and women doing the right thing, wrongly convicting an innocent person results in reduced trust in community leaders and authorities. A reduced trust can often lead to chaos and social disorder. Therefore, any crime should be proved beyond reasonable doubt, even if ten guilty persons escape.

Anti-theses: If a community would allow for ten guilty people to escape rather than wrongly convicting an innocent person to suffer, it will be bound to have many criminals in the street, escaping rightful judgement. To have a safe community, guilty persons must not escape, even if one innocent suffers.

Author's perspective: Affirmative

Title: Innocent until proven guilty

Ever since the first crime was committed, innocent men, women and children have suffered at the hands of criminals. The priority of any functioning community with the desire to have social cohesion would be to end the suffering of individuals which were upstanding citizens. Therefore, it is self-explanatory as to why punishing perpetrators for crimes committed have been of great importance in order to maintain social order. The safety and security of an innocent should be the prime concern of any community. To keep citizens safe is essential in order to encourage upright citizens to continue to refrain from crime. A justice system which wrongfully convict an innocent person will therefore have a greater detrimental effect on society than a justice system which have allowed ten guilty persons to escape.

The purpose of imprisoning guilty individuals is to protect innocent citizens from criminals. It would hold no purpose to prevent the escape of ten guilty individuals if the action did not reduce human suffering. In a hostage situation, negotiations are carried out extensively to prevent the suffering of innocent individuals irrespective of the number of hostages. If the individuals held hostage suffer at the hands of the guilty, the aim of the hostage situation is compromised. It is recognised in these hostage situations that allowing ten guilty people to escape is more humane than to allow innocent people to suffer. The suffering of a single individual defeats the aim of a justice system in keeping a community safe.

In 1948 the declaration of human rights was drafted to reiterate the sacredness of a human life. Preventing guilty individuals from escaping is meant to make the world a safer place, but it will serve no significance if the system is not prepared to trade innocent life for ten guilty people. In 2010 the Israeli government offered to trade a single Israeli soldier with a thousand Egyptian prisoners. From the perspective of the Israeli government, their soldier was innocent, and their prisoners were not. There are many would argue that the Israeli soldier is the guilty individual and this may be true. However, the offer made by the Israeli government expressed the value it places on its citizens and suggested that the trade for a single life they considered innocent was worth that off thousand prisoners. In fact, this move by the Israeli government indicate that it's better that not only ten, but even a thousand guilty persons then one innocent to suffer.

It is well recognised that the suffering of any innocent is not desired and should never be accepted. However, some would argue the importance of preventing guilty individuals from escaping punishment is more important than having innocent people suffer in order to maintain low crime rates and social order. However, if innocent people suffer at the hand of the justice system, its sole purpose of protecting its citizens is defeated. In the first gulf war, a coalition of 32 nations attempted to remove the Baath government from power in Iraq. However, the coalition did not initiate the removal of the government and allowed for the Baath to indiscriminately place their citizens through daily suffering. The Iraqi justice system would prove to be corrupt and would place the burden of individuals to prove their innocence when accused of guilt. This was particularly true if anyone was accused of collaborating with the enemy. The view the government held was that it was fine for innocent to face undeserved suffering if all guilty individuals were captured. This led to a society where fear was commonplace, and innocence was difficult to prove. Not surprisingly, the citizens did not place much trust in the authority and social cohesion deteriorated as a result.

Although not many ethical justice systems would support or allow guilty individuals to escape judgement, the entire purpose of the justice system is to protect the innocent. Based on such premise, it is of vital importance that no innocent person suffers for the justice system to be just, even at the expense of efficiency. In the circumstances where innocent people suffer, social cohesion and social order suffers, and communities deteriorate as a result as reflected by the examples in the essay. It is therefore important that no innocent person suffer, even if ten guilty persons were to escape.

"That some should be rich, shows that others may be rich, and hence it is just encouragement to industry and enterprise"
Abraham Lincoln

Definitions:

Rich: Wealthy in material possessions.

Encouragement: Providing support and confidence.

Industry and enterprise: Economic activity involving a collection of businesses and manufactures.

Thesis: In a capitalist society, wealthy individuals have the ability to encourage less wealthy individual to pursue economic ventures. This encouragement would also inspire less wealthy individuals to replicate the wealthy in the hope to stimulate an economy.

Anti-theses: Wealth is often passed down generations, and it is difficult for most individuals to move above the wealth bracket their parents were in.

Author's perspective: Affirmative

Title: The rich are encouragement to those who would like to be rich

 Since the dawn of human existence, citizens have worked very hard to make a living. Throughout history, there have always been a separation of social classes among those who have, and those who do not have. Such distinction between the rich and the poor was often criticised as being unfair and inhumane. However, visionaries like Abraham Lincoln suggested that wealthy individuals acted as an encouragement and reassurance for the less fortunate that they too may be wealthy. This type of thought pattern offered individuals with the incentive to think of creative ways to participate in both industry and enterprise and has been the cornerstone of the capitalism in the west for centuries.

During the second half of the 20th century, great economic progress and increased in wealth was seen in nations that adopted capitalism such as the USA in comparison to more centralised economies such as the Soviet Union which experienced economic collapse. In order for a nation to be prosperous, incentives were given for people to pursue industry and enterprise. This incentive in found in the western capitalist economies increased wealth and improved living standard. Abraham Lincoln explained that it was healthy for the economy to have a distinction between the wealthy and the average citizens as this offered less wealthy individual encouragement that wealth is achievable. This encouragement was not available in centralised economies as individuals did not own means of production, and wealth depended on the collective and not the individual. This provided much less incentive for the individual to work longer hours in the labour force, and such nations often depended on patriotism and other factors to encourage labour force involvement. Thus, based on historical economic growth, it can be seen that Abraham Lincoln was correct regarding a distinction in wealth being a great encouragement to both industry and enterprise.

Wealthy individuals are often responsible for job creation as they depend on labour for their enterprise. In return, less wealthy individuals benefit from the job creation provided by the wealthier. Individuals involved in private enterprise who are wealthy may not always be liked by those who are less prosperous, but that does not prevent the dependence between both individuals for work. This symbiotic relationship, although not universally cherished provides the less wealthy individuals with jobs and livelihood to provide for themselves and their dependants. It also gives many employees the encouragement to increase their wealth by realising that greater wealth is achievable by witnessing it personally. Although many argue that capitalism has plenty of flaws and that wealth difference among citizens can act as a catalyst for social division, it is difficult to argue that wealth division also offers great encouragement to industry and enterprise.

In nation's where few people are rich, industry and enterprise are often not encouraged. It is difficult to provide incentive for individuals to put greater effort into industry and enterprise when every citizen is caught in poverty except for individuals in power such as royalty, dictators or government officials. There probably is no greater discouragement than the lack of wealthy role models in non-government careers. The examples of such nations are plentiful ranging from socialist nations such as Venezuela to middle eastern nations such as Iraq and to African nations such as DRC. What these nations have in common is the widespread poverty and the centralisation of power and finances. The means of industry and labour is centralised, and the average individual will never be given the opportunity to pursue individual enterprise and industry without severe government intervention. Such distinction between those in power compared to those not in power can lead to social division and discouragement among ordinary citizens. In these economies, no ordinary citizens can pursue wealth and be free from government intervention, and therefore the only encouragement is to power and not to industry and enterprise Therefore allowing some to be rich without political power provides encouragement to industry and enterprise rather than revolutions and overthrow of current individuals in power.

In essence, it holds true that financial division among social classes leads to encouragement of both industry and enterprise. Although it must be recognised that the sane division can lead to resentment within the population, it remains an important driver for a healthy industry. This hypothesis is well supported by the historical economic growth of nations that adopted a less centralised economy and enabled individuals to be rich through industry and enterprise.

"The mother of Revolution is Crime and Poverty" Aristotle

Definitions:

Revolution: The forcible overthrow government or social order in favour of a new system.

Crime: An act which is considered illegal by the constitute a person is located in and which is punishable by law.

Poverty: Is a state having minimal or no wealth or being in a state of inferior quality.

Mother: The entity or source that gives rise to a new creation/society/individual.

Thesis: Social failures found in revolutions often stem from an incompetent governing body. A governing body which fails to provide for its citizens adequately provides the basis for a revolution. The inadequacies from poverty and crime against humanity have often been the main reasons for uprisings and revolutions of the past. Thus, it would be safe to say the state of poverty and acts of crimes should be labelled as the mothers of revolution.

Anti-thesis: Revolutions are often thought of as political acts and are not necessarily related to corruption. A large number of revolutions resulted in greater crime, corruption and reduced living standard. Famous examples include the communist revolution of Russia in 1917 and the Nazi revolution in Germany in 1933. These examples both highlight two systems where both crime and poverty increased both in frequency and poverty and required external factors to bring down the respective government of the time.

Position of author: Affirmative

Title: To overthrow the government, you first need crime and poverty

Since the dawn of human civilisation, revolutions have been utilised to replace governments to bring in a new social order. The fire of such revolutions has often been sparked by government failures and their inability to provide for the general public. Not being provided with wealth or safety, many citizens have no reason to ask or perhaps even actively pursuing a change in their governing bodies. Although it is true that many factors have contributed to revolutions of the past, no factors have been as potent as crime and poverty, the secret ingredients of even the greatest revolutions. So potent are both crime and poverty that even ancient historians like Aristotle recognised their influence and labelled them the "mother of revolution".

In every society there are issues which make citizens frustrated however, two particular issues that have people up in arms are crime and poverty. These two issues appear to be unforgivable in that they raid the nation of wealth and safety, providing citizens with little reason to not wish for change. Most notable contemporary examples where crime and poverty brought about a revolution is the African nation of Libya under Gaddafi. Libya was known to have vast natural resources, and yet the nation was plagued with citizens amidst poverty and rampant crime. Corruption and lack of planning by people in positions of power led to high levels of crime, poverty and in the aforementioned examples even civil war. Countries like Libya among others provide a good example on how a corrupt government limit the safety and wealth of its citizens and lead to a society full of crime and poverty. The Libyan revolution was justified for a large number of reasons, but it was evident that the mother of these reasons were high levels of crime and poverty.

Certain revolutions are often believed to be mainly due to nationalism and self-governance rather than crime and poverty. However, looking beyond the surface one can appreciate that although a nation may be relatively free from crime and poverty, certain groups within the nation may not enjoy the same privileges as the rest of the population. A notable example of such nation is that of the former republic of Yugoslavia in 1991. Yugoslavia was often thought of as a relatively peaceful and stable nation where levels of crimes and poverty were lower in comparison to most other nations. However, the majority of wealth remained firmly in the hand of the Serbian part of the population, and much less were granted for the people of Croatia, Slovenia and Macedonia. The non-Serbian population of Yugoslavia were experiencing much greater levels of crime and poverty, and it was not long until a revolution was in full motion and Yugoslavia was disintegrating into many different nations. Although this particular revolution did have a component of nationalism, and other political motives, the issues of crime and poverty were certainly strong underlying factors.

Several revolutions have also been waged against the ruling class by its citizens for the vast difference in wealth between the ruling class and the ordinary citizen. The poverty faced by ordinary citizens in middle eastern nation's where the ruling class have some of the world's wealthiest individuals in the world is nothing short of a crime against humanity. Several middle eastern nations had a change of rulers throughout the middle east in the last few years, and several more privileges have been offered to the working class. The governments of Yemen and Syria have been put to the test as their citizens no longer want to see their children die of starvation while watching their rulers enjoy all the luxuries of life. It appears that crime and poverty are not accepted by society and could naturally lead to a revolution.

Revolutions, or the forcible overthrow of status quo is result of a number of reasons however, crime and poverty is often the greatest drivers of revolution. Many motives can be attributed to initiate revolutions, but as in all the examples provided it is notable that the common denominator remains crime and poverty. It appears that although other reasons can act as powerful motivators however, in isolation these reasons remain mere motivators and will be unable to sustain a revolution. Therefore, it can be appreciated that as Aristotle suggest, crime and poverty are the source, or in other words the mother of revolutions.

Type B Essays:

"That man is the richest who's pleasures are cheapest" H.D. Thoreaus

Definitions:

Richest: The wealthiest individuals in terms of tangible and intangible goods.

Pleasures: An activity or object that provides satisfaction and enjoyment.

Cheapest: Most affordable object or activity.

Affirmative/Thesis: There is no limit to the cost of worldly pleasures. Some riches are without reach even for the world's most wealthy individuals and therefore to be truly rich, one's pleasure must be the cheapest.

Negative/Anti-theses: It is difficult to experience pleasure in an expensive world like today. To have cheap pleasures reflects limited wealth.

Author's perspective: Affirmative

Paragraph ideas:

1) Material wealth is only one aspect of richness.
2) Those who are wealthy may not be the happiest.
3) An important, but often neglected aspect of community wealth is social capital
4) Happiness has no price, and no amount of wealth can afford the most expensive pleasures. Therefore, a man is richest who's pleasure are the most affordable.

Since time- immemorial, both men and women have sought pleasures in all aspects of life. It is well known that not all share the same pleasures, and that some pleasure are more expensive than others. The materialistic wealthy may afford the more expensive pleasures, but often is those who are content with the simple pleasures in life that are truly rich. The gold an individual possess is only valued relatively to what their heart desires. Therefore, the man who has the cheapest pleasures are certainly the richest.

Materialistic wealth is only one aspect of richness and is often used as the sole scale of wealth in the western world. It is without doubt that it is the materialistic wealthy that can afford the more expensive pleasures in life however, not all pleasures are affordable even by the wealthiest individuals. There is a limit to how much anyone could possibly afford, and problems arise when the price of a person's wish list exceeds the cost one is capable of paying. This becomes worse if an individual has had the ability to afford expensive pleasures in the past. On the other hand, a person who has the cheapest pleasures can afford to have such pleasures at any time. Affording pleasures never becomes an issue, especially when those pleasures are free. That individual will be forever wealthy.

The world happiness report published by the UN always rank Scandinavian and other western nations as the happiest in the world. This score heavily depends on statistics such as financial wealth, educations, access to health care and gender equality. However, a happiness report that uses financial wealth as an indicator to happiness is inherently flawed. Often individuals in these nations have expensive pleasures that reach far beyond what you can purchase. This include pleasures such as tight knitted community, strong faith, sense of purpose as well as strong bonds with family members and friends. Pleasures that may be financially rich, but certainly not easy to come by in an ever increasing individualistic and isolated western world. African and middle eastern nations such DRC, South Sudan and Lebanon often rank very far down the list. However, immigrants from those nations often have a yearning to go home despite endless civil wars, extensive joblessness and lack of health care. This certainly support that despite hardship in these developing nations there are many pleasures which immigrant yearns for even though those pleasures may be considered the cheapest. One can only wonder how rich these immigrants would have felt whose pleasures were the cheapest had there been jobs, healthcare and peace in their home.

Citizens of western nations have amazing benefits that many individuals could only dream of. Advanced health care, social welfare, greater wealth and excellent education are only some of the perks of being a citizen of a developed nation. However, what is not included in the quality of life measurements are the less measurable indicators of richness. It appears that developing countries place a much greater importance in community and family before financial wealth. One of the many examples include the citizens of Lebanon where individuals worked on average twenty-five hours per week. This was not because they lacked job opportunities but rather to ensure they spent more time with family and participated in community activities. On the other hand, citizens of Scandinavian nations worked on average greater than forty hours per week, close to twice that of Lebanese citizens. Although Scandinavians are financially better of, it does not reflect other type of richness. Richness that many Scandinavians experience include being time-poor, marriage and family breakdowns, and higher suicide rate than nations in dire financial circumstances. Based on such comparisons, it appears that the citizens of Lebanon certainly have cheaper pleasures and certainly appear much richer for it.

Therefore H.D. Thoreaus may have understood that expensive pleasures may soon have a greater cost than just the price tag. It appears that the many sacrifices undertaken by individuals to afford the more expensive pleasures can often make a person very poor in every other aspect of their life. So thus, it certainly appears "that man is the richest who's pleasures are the cheapest".

"He who knows how to be poor, knows everything" - Jules Michelet

Definitions:

Poor: Lacking material wealth.

Everything: All-encompassing knowledge.

Thesis: The ability and acceptance to be poor in a material world by choice is to know that material wealth is only a means to an end, and nothing more. It is all that there is to know therefore "He who knows how to be poor, knows everything.

Anti-theses: To be poor is often a state which is imposed on a person, and to be poor is a state that is often force upon a person rather than a source of knowledge.

Author's perspective: Affirms the thesis

Paragraph ideas:

1) A person who knows how to be poor is not necessary financially poor and certainly not poor in knowledge.
2) To know everything includes to know that happy is not those who have the most, but rather those who are content with the least. Being materialistically wealthy can often be a roadblock to connect and understand people.
3) Being materialistically wealthy can often be a roadblock to learn and understand individuals and to possess the wisdom to empathise with others.
4) In order to gain wisdom, one needs to be emptied from wealth and anything else, that will prevent a person from knowing anything.

Poverty is often viewed as a situation in which individuals are defeated to a point almost beyond help. It symbolises weakness in society as well as a problem that is an everyday life experience for many. Although being poor is mostly thought of as a financial status, Jules Michelet refers to it very differently in the quote; "He who knows how to be poor, knows everything". A person whose humbleness and humility prevents their pride and earthly possessions from consuming their life as Michelet explains, knows everything.

One does not necessarily need to be poor in order to understand how to be poor, but one must have been in circumstances of poverty. An average person who has experienced poverty is better equipped than a millionaire who has been fed with a silver spoon, as their gratification would offer them a greater pleasure of life. If someone truly knows how to be poor, he or she will understand their purpose in life in a more complicated manner and therefore know more, if not everything about their life. This is because they will realise that happy is not those who have the most, but rather those who are content with the least.

Wealth is often a measure of success employed by the western world however, one could argue (as many do) that wealth is a great obstacle to inner peace and happiness. The western world of today has turned much more materialistic relative to previous centuries, and this has been seen as very costly for the individual by many. Whether it is measured by levels of greed or rising crime levels, it is undeniable that an increasing level of wealth have had a dramatic effect on people's values. The increase in number of abortions, increasing suicidal rates and a higher divorce rates are argued by many to be caused by this careless notion derived from excess wealth. This may seem like a moral argument, however great credit must be given to this argument as even though we have the resources to feed a starving world, we choose to place profit ahead of humanity. One of the main causes of letting the world starve is that we no longer know what it means to be poor.

To truly understand another person, we are told to imagine ourselves in their shoes. In fact, this holds true beyond understanding people. In a capitalist society such as Australia, citizens are awarded based on their efforts, however it still chooses not to penalise those who are unhealthy or disabled. Taxpayers contribute to Medicare and social welfare even if they don't benefit from such resources. Although it is not a voluntary act, ministers in government have enacted such laws as they understood the meaning of a wealthy society and therefore did not adapt to nature's law of survival of the fittest. Other ideologies such as communism and socialism are also built on this quote as they encourage equality between citizens at the cost pride and status in society. In the Soviet Union, educational and financial status was not meant to differentiate the salary of individuals. In theory, the government taught its people how to be poor during difficult times, and therefore teaching them how to be poor financially and in spirit. As a results, everyone supposedly had a better understanding of their neighbour's circumstances. This idea of being poor in spirit is also touched by several of the world religions including Buddhism and Hinduism which teach their followers that enlightenment is only possible when a person is detached from earthly possessions. In addition, Jesus of Nazareth also mentioned in the Sermon on the Mount that the kingdom of heaven belonged to those who are poor in spirit, referring to those who are empty of earthly desires. This notion of knowing everything through poverty in spirit and earthly objects has been shared throughout history and seems to be offered plenty of credential by different ideologies and religions. Although slightly different, all of these lessons teach that in order to gain such understanding, one needs to be emptied from anything that will prevent a person from knowing everything.

It seems very logical that a student of life can only succeed with an open mind and plenty of concentration. A person who understands what it means to be poor is free from such distractions. This idea of poverty offering enlightenment and a much greater understanding is not only shared by Michelet but has also been concluded by many great teachers of the past and taught throughout history through different ideologies and religions.

"I can usually judge a fellow by what he laughs at" – Wilson Mizner

Keywords: usually, judge, fellow, laugh

Definitions:

Usually: In most circumstances.

Judge: Make an opinion of something or someone.

Fellow: Another individual.

Laugh: The facial and bodily expression of joy and laughter.

Thesis: Laughter is to a large degree uncontrollable, and unlike spoken words cannot be easily manipulated. It acts as the unconscious revelation of someone's character.

Anti-theses: Laughter, like other expressions such as words and body language can be manipulated and acting skills can often disguise a person's true character.

Author's perspective: Affirms the thesis.

Paragraph ideas:

1) One's perception of a person depends on what they enjoy, and the way they react to a situation.
2) Laughter is often associated with happiness, joy and a high level of contentment. Such reaction enables an individual to judge a fellow by what he laughs at.
3) The level of intelligence can also be determined by what a fellow laugh at. Laughing at witty joke compared to laughter at a menial subject reveal plenty regarding a person's character.

4) Laughter is somewhat uncontrollable, unlike several other emotions.

Judging others based on the colour of their skin, attitude and clothing is an act that is carried out every minute of the day. Perceptions are made based on assumptions gathered by what is understood from our senses along with our own understanding of others. A person's own experience throughout life also comes to play when establishing perceptions. Therefore, it is difficult to correctly judge a person based on their acts, however a less controllable act such as laughter is a better indicator of who a person truly is. Wilson Mizner suggests that laughter is an act that he employs to build his perception of individuals and states that "I can usually judge a fellow by what he laughs at". An uncontrollable action which not only acts as an indicator of humour, but also one's contentment and level of intelligence

One is often told that there is more than one side of the story, and this can be attributed to the different way individuals observe the behaviour of the same person. Two people may witness the same scene at the same moment of time and still have a completely different perception of the individuals involved. There are numerous reasons as to why individuals, although seeing the same thing will perceive it differently. One of the reasons for different viewpoint being previous prejudices. No two people express their emotions in the same exact way, and that is why laughter, a somewhat uncontrollable act is a better indicator of a person's emotional status, level of enjoyment, and also one's contentment. Laughter is often an immediate reaction that is triggered without a conscience reaction. Therefore, it is fair by Mizner to say that "I can judge a fellow" by an act which does not constitute of a developed and conscience façade.

It takes a lifetime to completely understand another person, because it takes equally long to understand oneself. A witty person can easily put on a smile or play their poker face. Emotions seem to be uncontrollable, but some have greater control of their mood swings than others. Behind a smile might be a grave past, or dire circumstances. A façade full of tears might only be a game played as some individuals employ emotions as a hand of cards. Laughter is an expression of the soul screaming out its contentment, a mood far too difficult to sustain, and too difficult to reach in troubled times. Through extrapolation of Mizner's quote, a person's situation and their control of the situation can be judged by what a person laughs at. If one can laugh their worries away and recognise problems as part of life, the person is more likely to be of a strong personal character.

Intelligence is another factor that is judged by many. What a fellow laugh at will often indicate their understanding and knowledge of a topic. A popular cartoon "the Simpsons" is a perfect example where various political and religious references are made to entertain the older audience. Although children make a large proportion of the audience, they fail to laugh at some of the witty entertainment presented. What a fellow laugh at offers his/her audience a perception of their level of intelligence and understanding of the content and an insight into their thoughts and belief.

Although most actions lead to assumptions which in turn offer perceptions, it is laughter which often offers a more accurate judgement of a fellow. This is mainly due to laughter being a less controllable act and denies a person of time and conscience ability to wear it as a façade. Laughter as Mizner suggests usually offers a better judgement of the fellow than what they say or do.

"It is amazing how complete the delusion that beauty is goodness" – Leo Tolstoy

Keywords: amazing, complete, delusion, beauty, goodness

Definitions:

Amazing: An act or object which causes great surprise or wonder.

Complete: All encompassing.

Delusion: A belief held that is contraindicated by reality.

Beauty: Something that is pleasing to observe.

Goodness: Being morally right or virtuous.

Thesis: The view that beauty equates to goodness is propagated by the Hollywood industry and our senses. Experience however often tell us otherwise. Goodness and beauty do not have any correlation.

Anti-theses: The goodness of a person or an object often radiates out as beauty. A dish is often made tastier due to its beautiful presentation, rather than the lack of it.

Author's perspective: Affirms thesis

Paragraph ideas:

1) Attractiveness captivates the eye to a degree which hinders the brain from interpreting reality correctly.
2) Beauty is a poor measurement of goodness
3) Beauty is in the eye of the beholder, goodness on the other hand is less subjective.
4) Goodness is found everywhere, often in the last beautiful of places.

Title: The deception of beauty.

Too often individuals make the wrong association between beauty and goodness. Although the two are closely related in the world of Disney and Hollywood, in reality the two are often independent of one another. In truth, one only has to look outside the window to realise that beauty may be danger in disguise. The beauty of an unkindled force such as Niagara Falls or the charm of the devil's helmet is undeniable, but despite their beauty they remain no less deadly. Despite endless number of contradicting examples, the delusion that beauty is goodness still remains.

The breathtaking scenes of the jungle and waterfalls are captured in millions of photographs, and yet no one dares to step too close to either scene without precaution. The same goes for humans, especially those who we label beautiful. The attractiveness of a being often captivates the eye to a degree which hinders the brain from interpreting anything else but what is captured by the eye. Such captivation by beauty unfortunately enforces the delusion which is delightfully expressed by Leo Tolstoy: "It is amazing how complete the delusion that beauty is goodness".

Several years ago, I was in a relationship which was filled with nothing but goodness. Every minute of it was cherished and felt like the first. It was not until that my partner had been caught between two cars in a car accident that my life fell apart.

Although she had recovered, her beautiful face was filled with a number of scars. The first few months after the accident, things began to fall back into place, until the delusion became a burden too heavy to bear. No longer did she want a child or be near family or friends as she now thought she was no longer a good person. The endless stares from strangers completed her delusion that she was an outcast and made her believe that without her prior beauty she no longer belonged to the same society. I, along with friends and family tried to convince that she was still the same person, however, that delusion was far to complete. Soon she moved away and I have not heard from her ever since.

The delusion that beauty is goodness is only complete due to social stigma. The believe that perfection is attainable is underlined by a fallacy. It is the endless amount of make-up, the plastic surgery, anorexic Hollywood stars and models that contributes to such fallacy. Photoshop and visual techniques offer endless amount of fuel for the media to build upon the fallacy of perfection, and in the same time complete the delusion that beauty is goodness. The delusion is nothing but a anguish for those with unnerving levels of insecurity.

"Whether you think you can or you can't, you are right" – Henry Ford

Key words: can, can't, right

Definitions:

Can: The ability to do a certain action.

Can't: The inability to do a certain action.

Right: Being correct.

Thesis: A person's mindset often determines the outcome of an action. A person who believes they may be able to complete a task will set out to achieve a task despite all the obstacles faced. A person who believe they can't complete a task will cease any attempt when faced with any adversity.

Anti-theses: The outcome of a task is determined by someone's skillset and determination, and not what they believe. Many delusional individuals set out to do many tasks which they are certain they can do but never complete.

Author's perspective: Affirms the thesis

Paragraph ideas:

1) An individual's outlook often determines the outcome.
2) Will power, faith, self-confidence and determination is the difference between a winner and someone who quits.
3) First step of victory is possessing a victor's mentality.
4) A negative mentality is a draining when aiming for a favourable outcome.

Title: Result: Yet to be chosen

Since the dawn of human existence, many challenges have been faced by humankind. These challenges or obstacles have shaped the life of the earthly population in a large number of ways. In places and conditions thought to be non-viable, human have strived and excelled due to determination. The saying that states "where there is a will, there is a way has proved over and over again to be true. The mentality possessed is one of the most important factors in deciding the final result.

During the early years of my daughters schooling, she actively took part in the 50-metre race in the athletics carnival. A close friend of her, Sandra was often denied participation in the race due to her disability with a missing leg muscle since birth. A few years later, I was astonished at the fact that Sandra took part of the 100-metre race and refused to accept a handicap start. Even more astonishing was the fact that she won the race. Soon after the celebration she was asked as to why she had not taken the handicap to her advantage. To everyone's disbelief she replied that her advantage was that she had to try harder during practice. Her mentality had decided the results.

The importance of such mentality in deciding the outcome of a result is delightfully expressed by Henry Ford in his quote: "Whether you think you can, or you can't you are right".

Interestingly enough, Ford was often doubted when making an American automobile and was made the laughingstock of the vehicle industry. His determination led to great success over the continent, and the establishment of one of the largest automobile company today. His determination, and the believe that he could make the car led to his success. A more modern example is that of Barrack Obama, the first non-white president of USA. A milestone in history was achieved as an outcome of Obama's campaign of "yes we can" and the believe that he could achieve what he set out to do.

The true outcome of someone's mentality can work both ways. It can labour in a negative fashion if we doubt our own ability to achieve an outcome. In doubting, a self-fulfilling prophesy of failure begins to take place. By stating that we can't, we are doomed to fail.

Challenges are met every day. And the mentality and determination of an individual remains pivotal component in the final outcome of a result. Whether one think they can, or can't, they are often right, and we often choose our own results without even realising.

"You grow up the day you have your first real laugh – at yourself"   Ethel Barrymore

Keywords: first, real laugh, yourself

Definitions:

First: The initial.

Real laugh: Unforced laughter.

Thesis: The ability to be truly light-hearted and accept who you are is the day personal growth is possible. Until then, you are pretending to be someone else and will continue to do so until you truly accept who you are.

Anti-theses: Laughing at yourself indicate that you are not taking yourself seriously enough and is often a sign of weakness.

Author's perspective: Affirms the thesis

Paragraph ideas:

1) Being too serious can often be a hindrance to personal growth.
2) Taking oneself too seriously can often be hurtful and have a personal toll.
3) Realising the minor role an individual has inside the scope of the world can often become a great relief.
4) A humble life free from stresses is personal growth that can be derived from a humble mindset.

Title: Laugh, and you shall grow!

Since the dawn of time, human beings have always had the desire or wishful thinking that they themselves would acquire qualities which they did not possess. The desire to become stronger, more intelligent and to always be a step ahead has driven this world forward. Such mentality has contributed largely to where we are now. Although such desires make the human race more competitive, it also diminishes the purpose of life. Pride and fame drive people to the point of madness and prevent them from growing up. Without the gift of humility, one cannot grow up and understand the destructive force of pride. The only way to grow up and understand that life is not all about lingering on the past and wonder what you could have done differently is to really laugh at oneself.

Every person has a past, a fact which is simply undeniable. A person's past is only as destructive to oneself as it is permitted to be. The scope of negative memories from the past is only relevant in relation to the harm it poses on the individual. It is rather a person's ability to laugh at oneself that really enables them to be distant from the negative impacts of such memories, and in turn grows both emotionally and intellectually.

It is not a rare sight to see citizens roaming around the city with an emotionless expression on their faces. Too often it seems like the weight of the whole world rest on their shoulders. In Barrymore quotes, it seems that in order to grow up that one must realise the minor role one plays in the scope of the world, and that this entire world does not depend on an individual person. The ability to laugh at previous thoughts and framework of thoughts is what will enable one to grow up, maybe not physically, but certainly emotionally and mentally.

A large portion of the population is burdened by expectations, both personal and communal, in addition to the destructive nature of comparing oneself to others. The ability to de attach oneself from such burdens is a gift in itself and allows an individual to grow in character. The ability to laugh at oneself is the key to a simple and harmonious lifestyle which permits an individual to enjoy one's own past and presence. By simply laughing at oneself, an individual is given the key to a humble life, free from the stresses of expectations.

Challenge:

With the quotes below, attempt at planning an essay. With appropriate planning of each quote, attempt at a creative piece and have them reviewed by a friend who is also preparing for the GAMSAT for feedback.

Perhaps I know why it is man alone who laugh. He alone suffers so deeply that he had to invent laughter – Friedrich Wilhelm Nietzsche

Key Words:

Definitions:

Thesis:

Anti-Thesis:

1) Laughter is freedom and ultimate remedy.
2)
3)
4)

From the deepest desires often comes the deadliest hate – Socrates

Key Words:

Definitions:

Thesis:

Anti-Thesis:

    1)
    2)
    3)
    4)

Conform and be dull – J F Dobie

Key Words:

Definitions:

Thesis:

Anti-Thesis:

1)
2)
3)
4)

Hatred is the coward's revenge for being intimidated – G.B Shaw

Key Words:

Definitions:

Thesis:

Anti-Thesis:

    1)
    2)
    3)
    4)